DIY NATURAL HOMEMADE HAIR CARE

A handbook for all hair type

With 30 Recipes.

Johnson .c. Brown

Copyright

All Rights Reserved. Contents in this book may not be copied in any way or by means without written consent of the publisher, with the exclusion of brief excerpt in critical reviews and articles.

Table of contents

Chapter one...6

Introduction 6

Chapter Two 8

Natural home made Shampoos: 8

Home made coconut milk and honey

shampoo: 8

Home made chamomile /aloe vera shampoo 10

Home made rosemary shampoo...................11

Home made baking soda shampoo with aloe

vera 12

Home made lemon juice shampoo with olive

oil 13

Home made baking soda and lemon juice

shampoo..14

Home made aloe vera shampoo 15

Home made honey and vitamin e oil shampoo

....16

Home made rhassoul clay and honey 16

Home made honey shampoo and hempseed

oil 17

Home made egg and honey shampoo 18

Home made coconut milk and peppermint oil 19

Home made thyme and calendula shampoo .20

Home made lemon peel, plantain and rose petals...20

Chapter Three 22

Natural home made conditioners. 22

Home made lemon and egg conditioner 22

Home made banana and milk conditioner 23

Home made apple cider vinegar and honey leave on conditioner 24

Home made yogurt and jasmine oil...............25

Home made aloe vera gel and lemon juice conditioner..26

Home made coconut oil and rosemary water 26

Home made vitamin e and coconut milk conditioner..27

Home made almond and rose water conditioner..28

Home made yogurt and peppermint conditioner.................................28

Home made avocado and mayonnaise conditioner.................................29

Home made sweet almond and rose oil conditioner.................................30

Home made shea butter and avocado oil conditioner.................................30

Home made coconut milk and shea butter conditioner.................................31

Home made avocado and shea butter conditioner.................................32

Home made aloe vera and shea butter conditioner.................................33

Home made egg yolk and lemon juice conditioner.................................34

Chapter one

Introduction

Your hair is an expression of your beauty and style. These recipes will help to guide your steps on things you need, to make your hair product. And also, utilizing the ingredients present in our homes, these products can be made in fewer amounts in which you may purchase very few items of the recipe for your own homemade natural organic hair care.

Most of the chemicals used in salon can be tough on your hair and these chemicals reduce the natural quality of the hair however when these hash chemicals come in contact with your hair, your hair is prone to frequent breakage and all other hair damages, but with this home made natural organic hair care your hair will return to its natural state. However, it might take a little time to recover fully. Still constant use of the homemade natural products will help in performing wonders, and this homemade natural organic hair care will give you an excellent result without the damage. Own a shampoo, conditional, oil, and other home made natural hair products its fun being able to create it

your self aside from personal use; you may sell
them to your friends.

Chapter Two

Natural homemade Shampoos:

This homemade shampoo takes good care of your hair, and it's full of a natural nourishing element. In making your shampoo, you need to know the basics ingredients and the combination rules and being careful of some essential properties each component contains and use them creatively. Get a suitable and clean container of your choice, preferably a squeezable one, which will make it more comfortable while washing your hair.

Homemade coconut milk and honey shampoo:

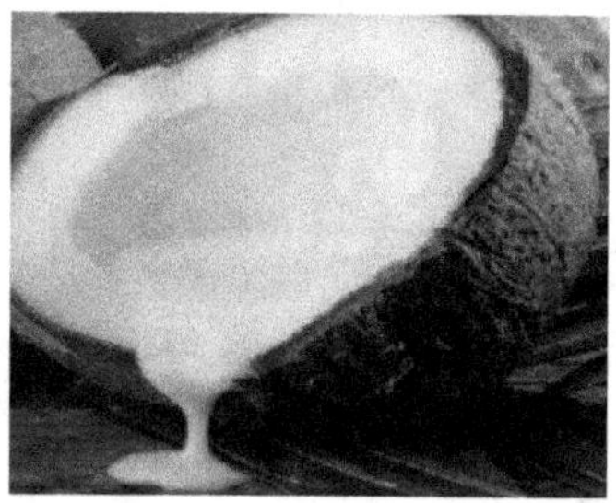

Ingredients:

- ¼ cup homemade coconut milk

- ¼ cup of liquid castile soap

- 15-20 drops of peppermint

- 30ml of honey

- ½ tablespoon of olive oil or coconut oil

Method:

Put the coconut milk in a clean bowl, pour the order into it and whisk until you get a good mixture and texture, shake well before each use.

Importance of the ingredient used to the hair.

Coconut milk: coconut milk is excellent for your hair. It is made from cracking the coconut and removing the flesh inside the coconut and blend with water, then sieved out; it is natural and contains essential vitamins like niacin and folate, which help the smoot flow of blood in the scalp. It contains vitamin E, B, and fats, which is important in fighting hair damage and all others; they also have a high protein profile that can keep your hair healthy.

Coconut oil is a natural oil that helps in restoring the natural health of the hair and as well to keep it shining.

Peppermint helps the hair grow fast and is essential in leaving your hair and scalp fresh and crisp.

Homemade chamomile /aloe vera shampoo.

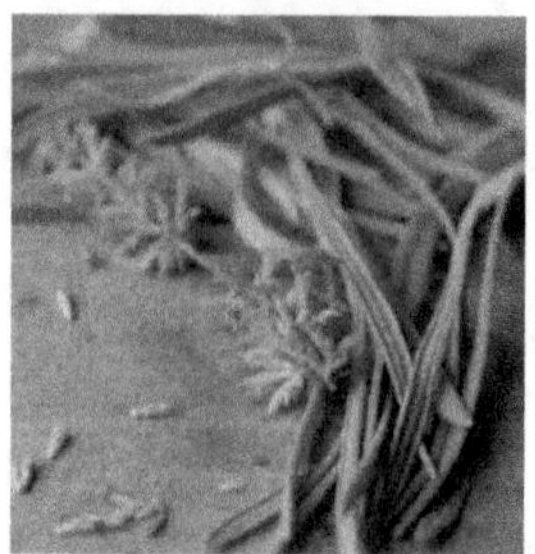

Ingredients:

- 2 cups distilled water

- 56.7g of dried chamomile

- ¾ liquid castile soap

- 2 tablespoons aloe Vera gel

- ½ teaspoon almond oil (omit for oily hair)

- 40-50 drops of tea tree essential oil

Method:

Boil the distilled water, and then add the dried chamomile in a low heat boil for 15 to 20 minutes, bring down from the heat and strain the chamomile from the liquid and dispose, then add the liquid castile soap and stir gently, add the aloe vera gel, almond oil, tea tree essential oil and stir well to get a good mixture, shake gently before each use

Homemade rosemary shampoo

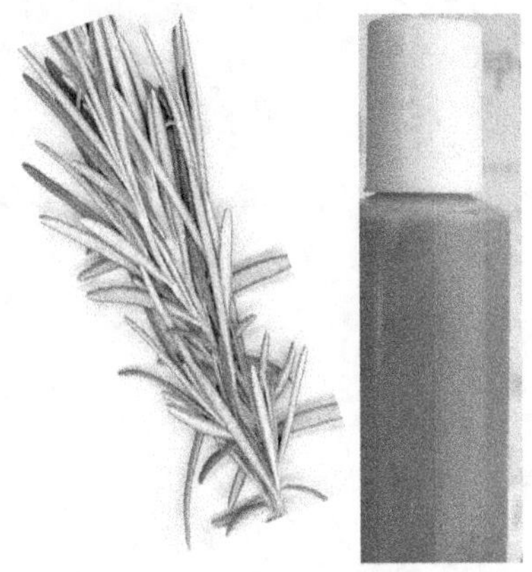

Ingredients:

- $^1/_4$ cup distilled water
- $^1/_4$ cup liquid Castile Soap
- 28g of dried rosemary
- 2 Tbsp. of olive oil
- 40-50 essential orange oil

Method

In a pot Boil the distilled water, add rosemary, and boil together for 10 minutes and strain the leaves and let it cool for a while, then add all ingredients to the boiled rosemary water and mix well by stirring.

Homemade baking soda shampoo with aloe vera.

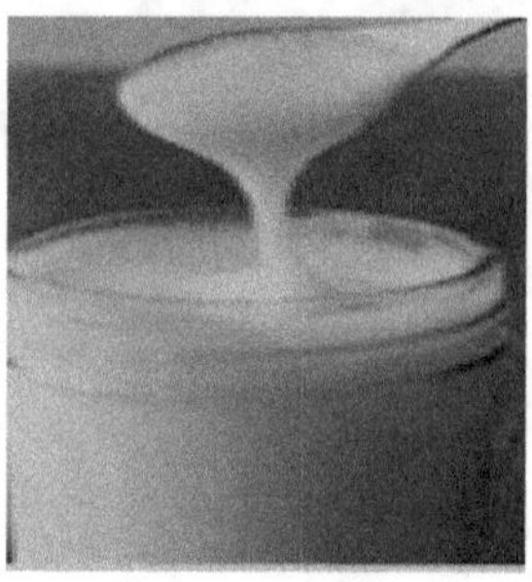

Ingredients

- ½ cup of baking soda

- ¾ cup of aloe vera gel

- 15ml of olive oil

- 20 drops of jasmine oil

Method

Place the baking soda on a clean bowl and add the aloe vera gel and mix properly then add the olive oil and jasmine oil stir till you get a good mixture.

Homemade baking soda shampoo with water

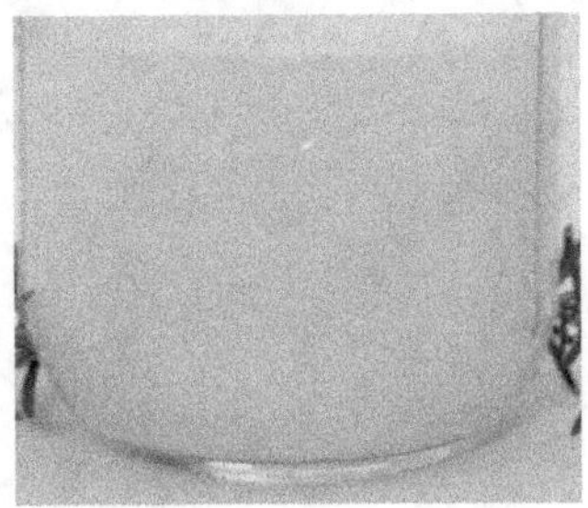

Ingredients:

- 1 cup of Distilled water
- 1/3 cup of baking soda
- 10 drops of lavender essential oil

Method:

Pour the distilled water in a clean bowl, then pour the baking soda gradually as you stir, add the essential oil, and make a good mixture, best stored in a bottled container.

Homemade lemon juice shampoo with olive oil.

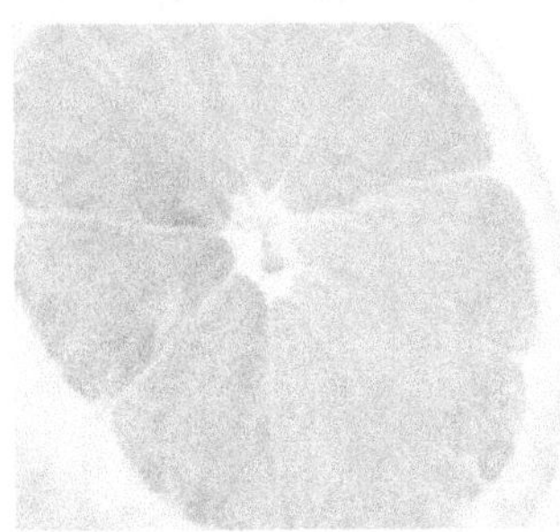

Ingredients:

- 15ml of olive oil
- ½ tbsp. Lemon juice
- 15ml of Fenugreek seed oil
- 2 drops of lavender essential oil
- ¼ cup of baking soda
- 2.5ml of apple cider vinegar

Method:

Mix the liquid content in a clean bowl and stir, then add the baking soda and stir.

Homemade baking soda and lemon juice shampoo

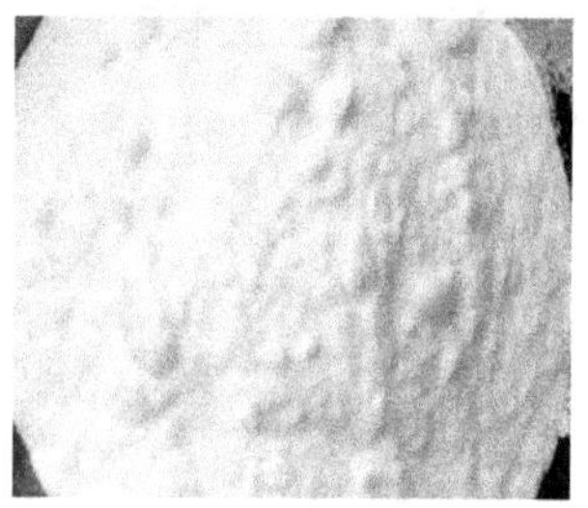

Ingredients:

- 2 cups of distilled water
- 30ml of Lemon juice

- 1TBS of baking soda

- 5 drops of Jasmine oil

Method:

Get a clean bowl and pour all the ingredients together stir correctly and store in a shampoo bottle

Homemade aloe vera shampoo

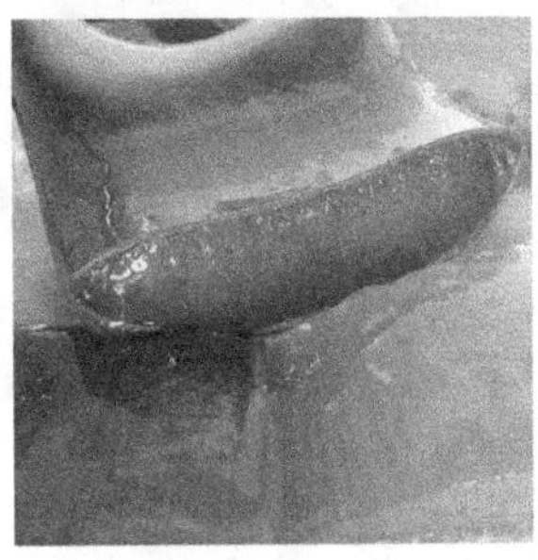

Ingredients:

- 2tsp of aloe vera

- ½ cup of liquid castile soap

- ¼ tsp of vitamin E oil

- 10 drops of lavender essential oil

- 1-2 tbsp. distilled water

Method:

In a clean bowl, mix castile soap and aloe vera juice stir and add vitamin E, essential oil, top with distilled water, store at room temperature.

Homemade honey and vitamin e oil shampoo

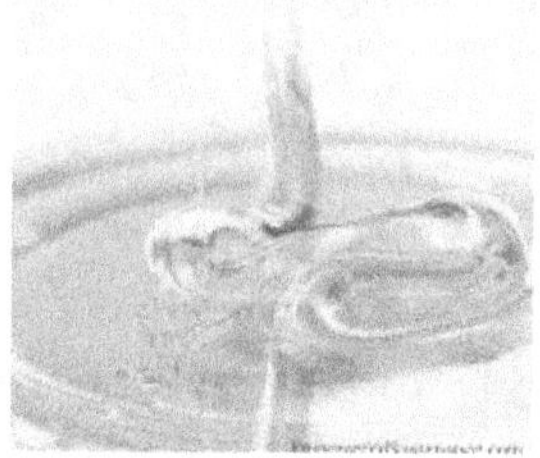

Ingredient:

- 3tbsp of natural honey

- 2tsp vitamin E oil

- 3 drops lavender essential oil.

Method:

Simply get a bowl put the natural honey, vitamin E oil, and essential oil together stir to form a paste, use every time you are going to shower.

Homemade ghassoul clay and honey ingredients:

- ¼ cup of distilled water

- 3tsp ghassoul clay

- 1 egg

- 4tsp honey

- 3 drops orange essential oil

- 1 tsp of avocado oil

- 7 drops of Jasmine oil

Method:

Pour the water, clay, egg, honey, avocado oil, Jasmine oil in a blender and blend for 7 seconds, it will show a foamy mixture then pour out in a clean bowl and add the essential oil and stir, store in a jar.

Homemade honey shampoo and hempseed oil

Ingredients:

- 3 tbsp. natural honey

- 1tbsp hempseed oil

- 3 drops lavender essential oil

Method:

Mix up all the above component and apply on the scalp.

Homemade egg and honey shampoo

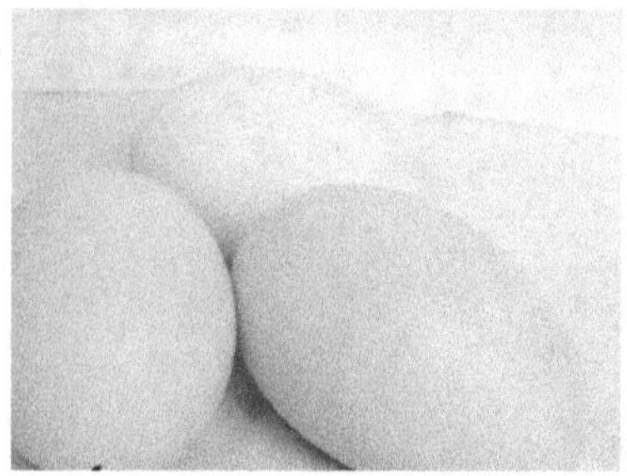

Ingredients:

- ¼ cup of distilled water

- 1 egg

- 2 tbsp. natural honey

- 2 tbsp. fresh aloe vera gel

- 8-10 drops of grapefruit essential oil

- 1 tbsp. of olive oil

- 5 drops of tea tree essential oil

Method:

pour all the ingredients in a speed blender and blend or whip till you get a good mixture.

Homemade coconut milk and peppermint oil.

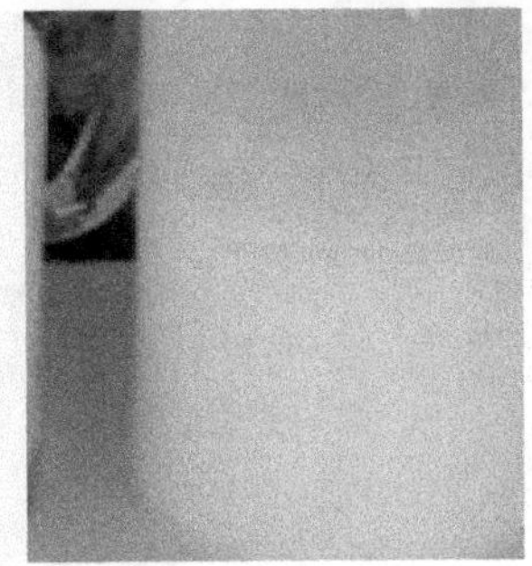

Ingredients:

- ¼ cup of coconut milk

- ¼ liquid castile soap

- 1 tsp vitamin E oil

- ½ tsp raw honey

- 10 drops of essential peppermint oil

Method:

Get a blender and pour the coconut milk, liquid castile soap, vitamin E, raw honey, and the peppermint oil into it and blend for 5 seconds and pour into a safe container.

Homemade thyme and calendula shampoo.

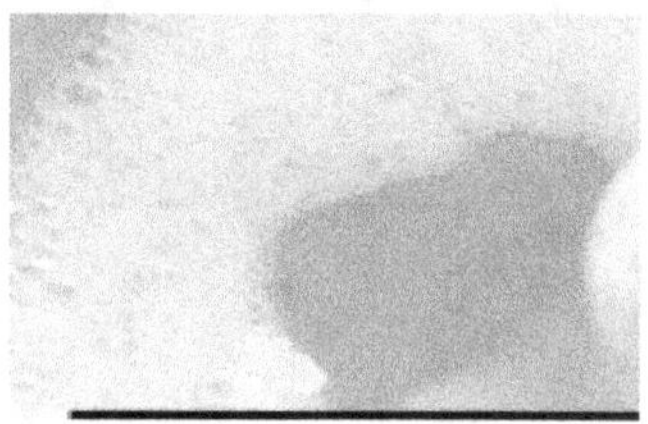

Ingredients:

- 28g of dried thyme

- 28g of calendula flowers

- 1/3 cup of mild castile soap

- ¼ tsp jojoba oil

- 15 drops of rose essential oil

- 10 drops of spearmint essential oil

- ½ cup of distilled water

Method:

Boil the distilled water, add dried thyme and calendula for 10 minutes, bring down to cool, strain the leaves and add up the remaining ingredients and stir.

Homemade lemon peel, plantain, and rose petals

Ingredients:

- 1 cup of distilled water infused with lemon peel, plantain, and rose petals
- 1/3 Dr. Bronner's castile soap
- ¼ tsp almond oil
- 10 drops of tea tree oil
- 5 drops of essential rosemary oil
- 15-20 drops of lemon essential oil

Method:

Strain the leaves out and dispose of the residue add the castile soap into the filtrate and stir then add up the others and mix properly

Chapter Three

Natural homemade conditioners.

This home made conditioner is rich in vitamins and minerals, which helps in rebuilding damaged hair to leave your hair beautiful. And makes it shinier, it helps in increasing hair elasticity and also reduces hair tangling. It is also useful in boosting moisture on dry hair, making it softer.

Homemade lemon and egg conditioner

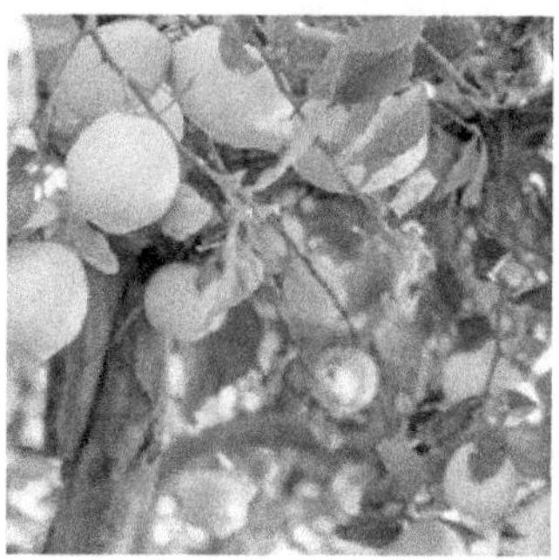

Ingredients:

- 2-3 eggs
- 2tbsp of lemon juice
- ½ tbsp. of jojoba oil
- 1tbsp of honey 1tbsp of vinegar

Method:

Get a bowl or better a blender, break the eggs into it and whisk, then add the other ingredients and mix well to form a paste, apply on hair for 10 minutes and rinse off with water.

Homemade banana and milk conditioner

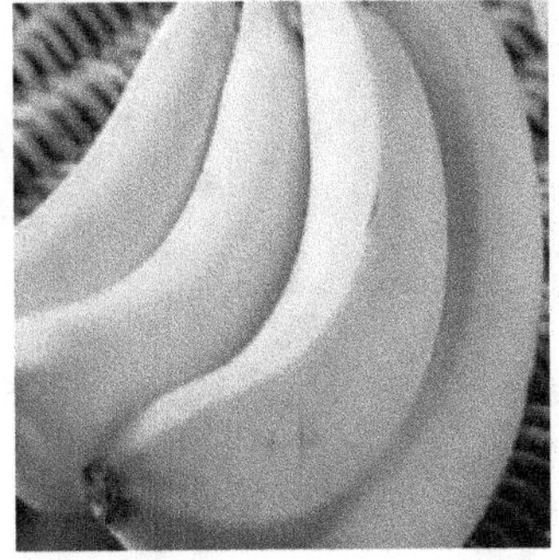

Ingredients:

- 2-3 banana
- 2-3 tbsp. of milk
- 2 tbsp. of honey
- 1 egg
- 2tbsp. of jojoba oil

Method:

Pill off the banana and put the soft part on a plate, put the other rest of the ingredient into a blender, and blend for a while, then put the banana into it and blend to form a paste, apply on hair for 15-20 minutes and rinse off with water.

Homemade apple cider vinegar and honey leave-on conditioner

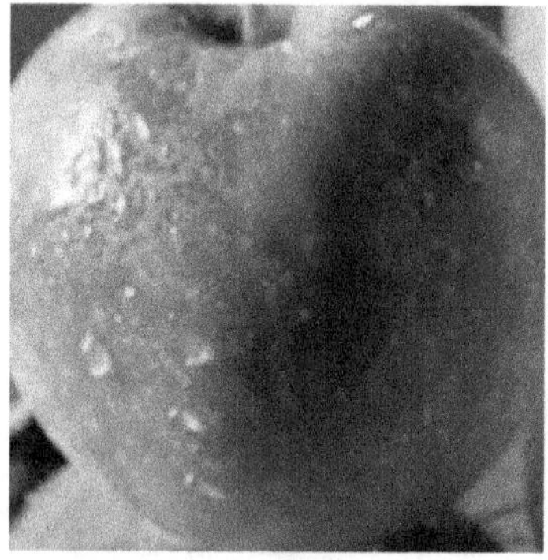

Ingredients:

- 4 tbsp. apple cider vinegar
- 2 tbsp. of natural honey
- 3 cups of water as a diluter

Method:

In a clean bowl, pour the ingredients into it and mix well, on a washed and clean hair pour on the hair tips, and do not rinse it.

Homemade yogurt and jasmine oil

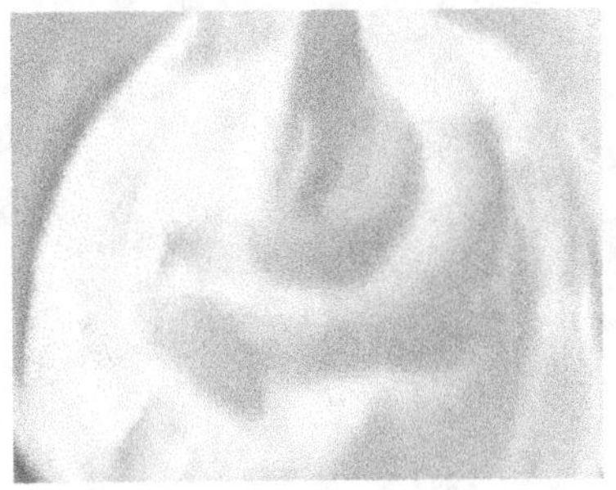

Ingredients:

- 6-8 tbsp. of yogurt

- 1 egg

- 5 drops of essential jasmine oil

Method:

In a clean bowl, break the egg into it and whisk, then add the yogurt and other ingredients and mix properly, apply on a clean washed hair for 15 minutes and rinse off with water.

Homemade aloe vera gel and lemon juice conditioner

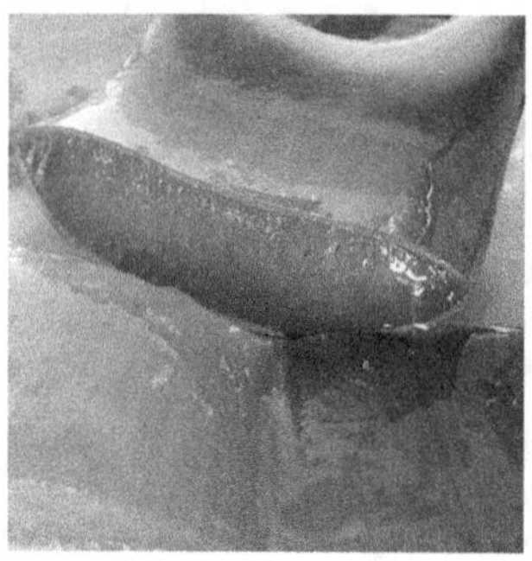

Ingredients:

- 5 tbsp. of aloe vera gel
- 1 ½ tbsp. of lemon juice
- 5 drops of lavender essential oil

Method:

In a clean bowl, mix properly and apply on shampooed hair for 10 minutes and rinse off with warm water.

Homemade coconut oil and rosemary water

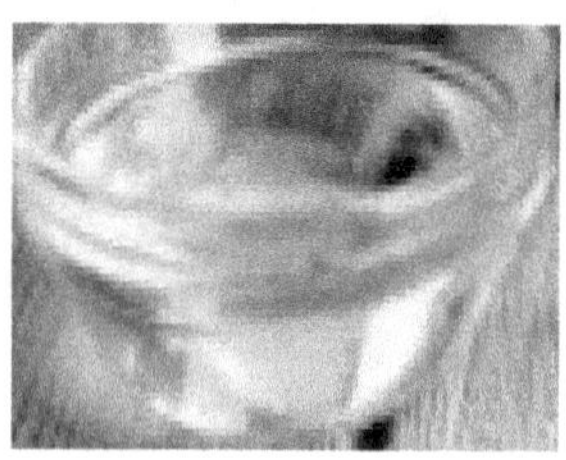

Ingredients:

- 2tbsp. of curd

- 1tbsp.o honey

- 1 tbsp. of rosemary water

- 1 tbsp. of coconut oil

- 1tbsp of lemon juice

Method:

Pour into a bowl all the ingredients and mix properly and apply on shampooed hair and leave for 10 minutes, then rinse off.

Homemade vitamin e and coconut milk conditioner

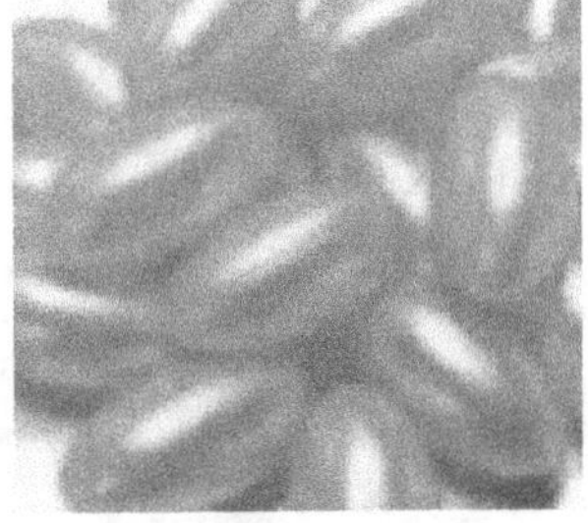

Ingredients:

- 2 capsule vitamin E

- 4 tbsp. coconut milk

- 2 tbsp. honey

- 1 tsp of rose water

- 1tsp of olive oil

Method:

Mix the ingredients properly on a bowl and apply on the scalp and hair, cover the hair with plastic cap steam the hair for 10 minutes to become soft and moist then rinse off with lukewarm water.

Homemade almond and rose water conditioner

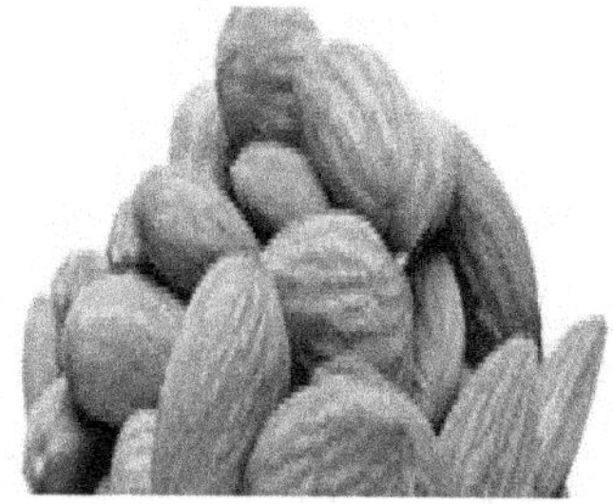

Ingredients:

- 1 tbsp. of almond oil
- 2tbsp of honey
- 2 tbsp. of coconut milk
- 2 tbsp. of milk
- 2 tsp of rose water

Method:

In a bowl, whip the ingredients and apply on shampooed hair for about 5 minutes and rinse off with water.

Homemade yogurt and peppermint conditioner

Ingredients:

- 5 drops of peppermint essential oil

- 4 tbsp. yogurt

- 1 tsp of coconut oil

- 1 tsp of honey

- 1 tsp apple cider vinegar

Method:

Stir in a bowl, add all the ingredients to form a good mixture apply on an already shampooed hair for 15 minutes and rinse off with lukewarm water.

Homemade avocado and mayonnaise conditioner

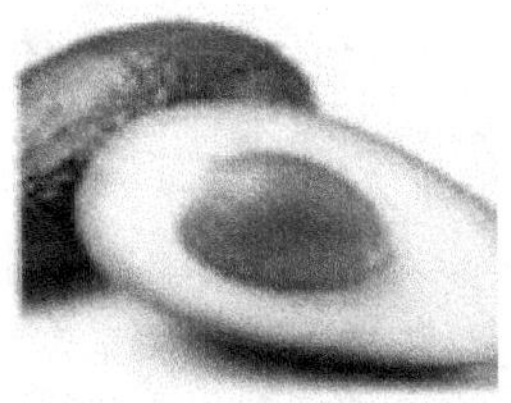

Ingredients:

- 2 avocado

- 1 cup of mayonnaise

- 5 drops of peppermint essential

- ¼ cup of distilled water

Method:

Peel off the back of the avocado and put the soft part into a blender then add the mayonnaise and the oil and blend to mix correctly, apply on a shampooed hair and cover with a shower cap for 20 minutes and rinse off with lukewarm water

Homemade sweet almond and rose oil conditioner

Ingredients:

- 1 cup of distilled water
- 2 tbsp. of sweet almond oil
- 10 drops of rose essential oil
- 1 tbsp. of guar gum

Method:

In a clean bowl, pour in the ingredients, and stir properly to avoid clumps, apply on the hair for 10 minutes and rinse with lukewarm water.

Homemade shea butter and avocado oil conditioner

Ingredients:

- 1 tbsp. shea butter
- 1 tsp of avocado oil
- 2 tbsp. of coconut oil
- ½ lemon juice

- 2 drops of spearmint essential oil

- 5-7 drops of jasmine essential oil

Method:

Use a microwave to melt the shea butter and the coconut oil together and allow it to cool until solid, then add the other ingredients and stir appropriately until creamy, your shea butter conditioner is ready.

Homemade coconut milk and shea butter conditioner

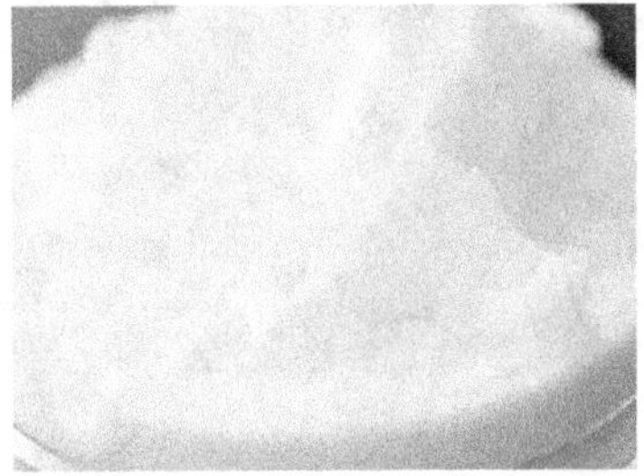

Ingredients:

- 1 cup of coconut milk

- 1 tbsp. shea butter

- 1 tsp argon oil

- 7 drops of tea tree essential oil

Method:

Pour in the coconut milk in a blender, shea butter and argan oil, blend for some seconds to form creamy then pour into a container and add the essential oil into it and stir properly

Homemade avocado and shea butter conditioner

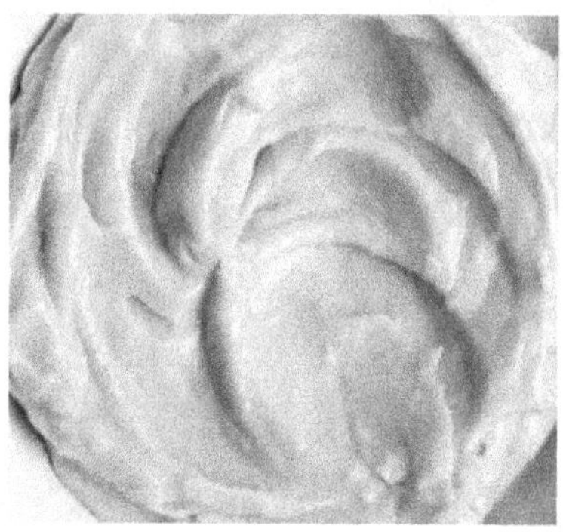

Ingredients:

- 2 avocado
- 1 tbsp. honey
- 1 tbsp. of shea butter
- 1 tsp of olive oil
- 5 drops of lavender essential oil

Method:

In a blender, blend the avocado, honey, shea butter and the olive oil to cream then pour into a container and add the essential oil and whip, this save as a deep conditioner

Homemade aloe vera and shea butter conditioner

Ingredients:

- ¼ cup of shea butter
- 1/3 cup of aloe vera gel
- 2 tbsp. Of jojoba oil
- 5 drops of lavender essential oil

Method:

Whip the shea butter using a hand mixer an add up the aloe vera as you mix to smooth cream

Homemade shea butter and Jiang Yiang oil conditioner

Ingredients:

- 2 tbsp. of shea butter

- ¼ cup of coconut oil

- 2 tsp olive oil

- 10 drops of yiang yiang essential oil

- 6 drops of peppermint essential oil

Method:

In a microwave, melt the shea butter and coconut oil, allow to cool, then add the olive oil, yiang yiang essential oil and peppermint essential oil, and stir properly.

Homemade egg yolk and lemon juice conditioner.
Ingredients:

- 2 egg yolk

- 1 tsp of fresh lemon juice

- 1 tsp vinegar

- 5 drop of lavender essential oil

Method:

In a blender pour in an egg, vinegar, lemon juice and blend until it takes the texture of mayonnaise, pour into a clean container and add the essential oil and whip, this save as a deep conditioner apply to hair and cover with a plastic shower cap for 10 minutes wash with cold or lukewarm water.